Brainstorming

Sophie Dallaway

ISBN: 1518741347
ISBN-13: 978-1518741340

Thank you to everyone for participating for
this photograph.

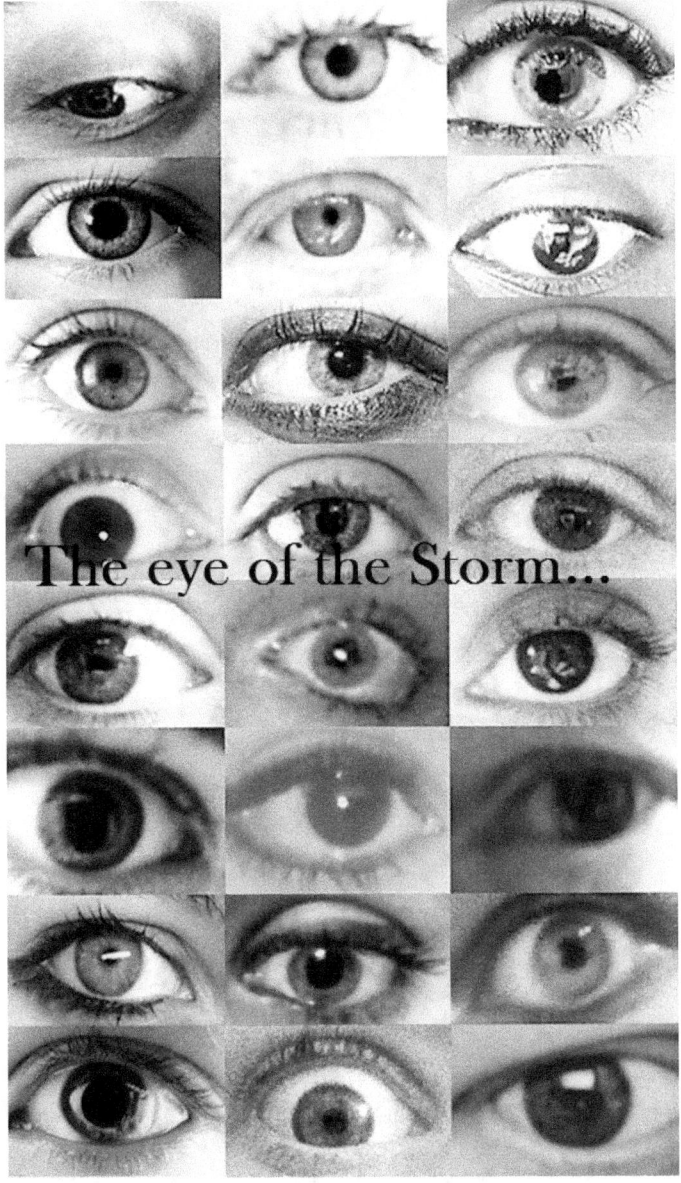

The eye of the Storm...

All conditions featured in Brainstorming have different severities; these are some examples or experiences and are not stereotypical.

"Come on and pull up a chair, 'cuz someone else's problems are worse out there, so cheers to the lot, so cheers to you lot." – Lena Lottie
(Cheers to the Lot)

CONTENTS

SNOW FOOTPRINTS

Buses, cars and lorries meet,

Compressed on the roads, hence why I

took the street;

Walked in inches, for miles; it was at

least over an hour,

Yet I powered through this snowy

shower.

I phoned religiously to say I was

running late,

But I would be there, no doubt, just

patiently wait.

Eventually I turned the corner; my

uniform was damp,

I brushed the snow off as I stepped up
the ramp,

I noticed something glint; something
important to discard,

I pulled it from the snow to reveal a
worker's security card.

I stormed and swiped in all the doors'
codes,

Burst in and blurted 'This was by the
roads!'

This monster shot through me, venom
hissed out of my mouth,

As I gave this sudden lecture I snarled
at the woman sitting south.

She looked half-witted, identical on
the tag,

When I asked to produce her card, she
rummaged in her bag;
'I haven't got it' Her mouth opened;
looking at my hand,
Eventually I handed over the card after
my overruling command.
Marching back to the station, the
demon disappeared,
Escaped out from my mouth then
whispered in my ear:
"Don't worry, I'm an aura, I'm here to
stay"
I shook my head and laughed, 'just go
away'
Several minutes later, I reached my
station at work,
A round of applause I was greeted

with; I thought they'd go berserk.

"It's snowing; the student's haven't come in today"

I felt triumphant in knowing I'd come such a long way.

Just moments later, I collapsed to the floor;

Drinks of tea from the staff; concerned as I did it more.

Eventually I was taken home, hearing phrases of 'get you on the mend'

But all I heard inside my ear was, "Hello, my new friend"

MORGAN'S SHOES

❖

"It's the fifth of March." Morgan sighed, looking at her calendar. She had crossed yet another day off with her black marker pen and placed it back down onto her desk full of teddy bears and dolls. "My birthday's tomorrow!"

Morgan looked out of her window and stared at the birds sitting on the top of the highest trees.

"I wish I was a bird." Morgan pouted, "I could do whatever I wanted then." she jumped onto her bed and splayed out her arms. The eight year old didn't like her birthday, in fact, she dreaded the very word!

When Morgan was six, she was diagnosed with a certain type of epilepsy called photosensitivity, which meant frequent, intense flashing lights and certain patterns would trigger a seizure.

"Morgan, dear!" her mother knocked, opening her door slowly.

"What, Mum?" she sat up, staring at her mother, who was smiling.

"It's a special someone's birthday tomorrow!" she announced enthusiastically; she sat next to

Morgan, who was looking dismal, and placed her hand on her knee. "Look, I know you aren't too excited, but it is *your* special day. You are a very special person Morgan!" she gave her a kiss on her forehead before returning downstairs.

"Urgh!" Morgan groaned, falling back on the bed again. She felt utterly empty and looked back out of the window at the birds; she wished she was able to soar free and glide past the trees into the sky and enjoy the warm flickering sun too.

The doorbell rang and it was Aunt Patricia and Uncle Dennis. They had brought two big bags for Morgan and handed her a purple envelope.

"Now, don't you open this until tomorrow!" Aunt Patricia told Morgan. Aunt Patricia was Morgan's favourite Aunt in the whole wide world; she was the kindest, most caring woman and always knew how to make her feel better when she felt blue.

"I won't." Morgan smiled, trying to peek inside the bags. Her father and Uncle Dennis were whispering and so were Aunt Patricia and her mother. Morgan tried to listen, but she couldn't work out what they were saying and before she knew it they were gone.

The next visitors were Grandma Rosie and Grandpa Joseph. Grandpa

Joseph propped his walking stick up against the wall and hung his jacket on the coat peg.

"Grandpa!" Morgan shouted as she ran to give him a massive hug. Grandpa Joseph looked at Morgan and ruffled her long blonde hair as he laughed.

"Look what your Grandma and I have for you! I know you've got a lot of presents to open..." he said, "But save the best 'til last!" he winked and handed Morgan a long parcel with silver wrapping paper and an envelope sellotaped to the top. Morgan let out a grin; her grandparents always got her the most extraordinary and wonderful presents.

Grandma Rosie turned towards Morgan and handed her a photograph; the photograph with worn edges was of a young girl around her age.

"Who's this Grandma?" Morgan asked, studying the girl with long wavy hair, holding an award.

"That girl, Morgan, is me!" she smiled, showing a few wrinkles. "I was a dancer when I was your age and a very good one too!" she looked reminiscent and turned the photograph over to reveal a note that somebody had handwritten in blue biro.

'Dear Rosie, My little dancer, Love from Mother x'

"That was from Great Grandma Beatrix!" Morgan exclaimed.

"It was indeed!" Grandma Rosie laughed, "Those, what I'm wearing in the photograph, were her dancing shoes. You see, she was a very talented dancer and quite well known too!"

Morgan sat up and her eyes grew wide as she was desperate to hear more about Great Grandma Beatrix.

"She was so elegant and graceful and everyone would watch her; the piano would play, she would dance and the audience would roar. It was marvellous!"

"I would have loved to have seen her, Grandma." Morgan stared at the photo of the girl holding the award decorated in ribbon, "But this is you!" Morgan instantly remembered.

"Exactly. Your Great Grandma passed down her dancing shoes to me and I became a great dancer too- that was my award for the best dancer in nineteen fifty-one, when I was your age!"

Morgan's mother overheard the conversation and smiled, looking at the photograph.

"Oh that old thing!" she laughed, "Your Grandma was one of the very best, Morgan!" Morgan placed the photograph onto her desk and smiled. She wished to be exactly like her

Grandma and her Great Grandma Beatrix.

Suddenly Morgan frowned and bit her lip and imagined a great big stage with thousands of luminous lights; flashing and changing at different speeds at different times.

"It's impossible." she sulked. Again, just before Grandma Rosie and Grandpa Joseph left, her mother and father were whispering. Morgan cupped her hand around her ear yet she still could not hear a thing.

Frustrated, Morgan sat on the sofa, crossed her arms and huffed,

"Why are people always whispering?" she thought, looking

outside the window, watching her grandparents get into their red car before tootling down the road.

Auntie Megan was the next to visit with Uncle Henry and Cousin Sam, followed by the neighbours: Thomas and Judy with their beloved cat, Oscar. Next, the doorbell rang with Melissa, Emily and Alice, who were Morgan's best friends; everyone had brought presents in all shapes and sizes, which were just impossible to guess; Morgan was a very lucky and loved girl.

Later that evening, Morgan was ready for bed. She took her medication and headed to her bedroom; as she tucked her duvet around her, she picked up the photograph once more and smiled, looking at Grandma Rosie's black sparkly shoes, and before she knew it she was fast asleep.

"HAPPY BIRTHDAY!" her parent's shouted. Morgan shot up out of bed; her hair was stuck to her face as she rubbed her eyes. She saw her mother holding a chocolate cake with birthday candles poking out of the top.

"Urgh!" Morgan groaned staring outside at the blazing sun. Again she saw the birds in the trees and, just like every ordinary day, she wished to be just like them.

"Here!" her father said. He had a huge grin on his face; he nudged a tiny green box towards her and watched as she opened it.

"It's a diary with some gel pens!" Morgan smiled. She opened the first page and read a note that was written in her father's handwriting:

'Write down all of the fun things you CAN do in here, not the things you can't. Love Mom and Dad x'

Morgan read those words and they played over and over in her mind throughout the day; suddenly she noticed he was right. Focusing on the positives made things easier than dwelling on the negatives. Just because there were things Morgan couldn't do didn't mean she couldn't do anything at all! There were still hundreds of things to do and hundreds of pages to fill.

Morgan leapt out of bed and gave her parents a tremendous hug.

"Thanks, Guys!" she looked out of the window once more and realised that birds couldn't do everything either; what she did realise was how happy they were with what they could do and how they embraced that.

"No one is perfect, but if they were, there would be nothing to achieve or sit and wonder about ...it would make life very boring." she thought with a smile.

It was time for Morgan to take her epilepsy medication again; she wished she could have a day off, considering it was her birthday, but annoyingly enough she had to take her tablets twice a day in order to stay controlled. This still meant she had to stay away from certain lights and patterns though, which was the reason why her face was still a little sad.

As she ran to the living room, Morgan saw the array of marvellous gifts from everyone who had visited her yesterday.

"This means no one will come today!" Morgan looked towards her mother, who was collecting a few cups in the kitchen.

"You said you didn't like birthdays, Morgan!" she replied looking at the birthday girl's troubled face. She then returned back to the kitchen.

"I don't feel like opening my presents." Morgan sulked. She hung her head and walked back upstairs; she wished she had appreciated her birthdays more. Morgan shut her eyes tight and hugged her pillow.

An hour passed by before the doorbell rang out. The sound made Morgan open her eyes and she heard it for the second time; she sprung up and slid down the stairs and opened the door.

"SURPRISE!" everyone shouted. Morgan was startled. There in front of her were: Aunt Patricia, Uncle Dennis, Grandma Rosie and Grandpa Joseph, Auntie Megan, Uncle Henry and Cousin Sam, Thomas and Judy, the neighbours with Oscar the cat and her best friends: Melissa, Emily and Alice!

"Come on through!" Morgan's mother beckoned; the living room was set out and decorated with balloons and a buffet that was full of savoury snacks and ice-cream, not to mention a wonderful chocolate Birthday cake.

They all sang Happy Birthday as Morgan opened her presents and she couldn't be happier; her smile got wider after she opened each card and present.

After everyone had eaten, they were starting to get a little tired and they were all ready for bed; it had been a great day for Morgan and she then knew what all the whispering was about! Her parents appreciated and understood how low Morgan's moods could be and decided a surprise would make her feel better and lift her mood.

When everybody had finally left, Morgan stood in front of Grandma Rosie and Grandpa Joseph with her silver wrapped present.

"You told me to save the best 'til last" she giggled. She excitedly ripped it open and watched the paper explode everywhere until it unveiled the gift inside. "What is it?" Morgan asked, looking perplexed. It was an old grey tarnished box; she placed it on the ground as her mother, father and grandparents gathered around her.

Morgan gripped the sides of the lid and pulled it upwards.

Mother and Grandma Rosie smiled, looking down at Morgan, until she let out a loud gasp.

"It's the dancing shoes!" she jumped up with the box for everyone to see how well the shoes still glistened; they were as beautiful as they were in the picture, if not more so, and they certainly were in marvellous condition. Hundreds of diamonds shone as the light caught them, making them so mesmerising and enchanting. "I shall be just like you and Great Grandma Beatrix!"

"Not only us!" her grandma replied "There's another picture inside the box…"

Morgan pulled out another photograph, which seemed a little newer than the one she placed on her desk; it was of a girl with brown hair taking a bow in exactly the same shoes. She turned the photograph around to see yet another handwritten message:

'From me to thee! Love you lots, Mom

x'

Morgan looked at the photo and realised immediately that the girl's features were her mother's.

"You were a dancer too, Mum?" she looked shocked; imagining her with a tutu, dancing on the stage in front of an audience.

"Oh yes, dear! A very good one just like your Grandma and Great Grandma!" she smiled, looking at the baffled birthday girl with the photograph in her hand.

"Why did you give it up?" Morgan looked at the photo, wondering why such a talented dancer would give up such a thing.

"Because after years I decided I wanted to be a mother." she ruffled Morgan's hair playfully and chuckled, "I told you, you're a very special girl! They've been in the generation for years and now we're giving these to you now Morgan. Happy Birthday!"

Morgan gave Grandma Rosie and Grandpa Joseph such a warm hug before they left and thanked them for a wonderful birthday; as they approached the door, Grandma Rosie held back and looked Morgan in the eyes and asked her why she looked sad.

"I will never get to be able to be a

great dancer like Great Grandma Beatrix, you or Mum." Morgan looked down at the wonderful shoes and remembered the vision she had with the stage and lights. "I couldn't because of the lights. I have epilepsy."

Grandma Rosie pulled in towards Morgan, smiled and whispered with a smile, "It didn't stop your Great Grandma Beatrix, did it?" Morgan looked quizzically. "She loved to dance but she too had photosensitivity, just like you, but that didn't stop her! She started dancing in her local town, in the old bars with the pianos; she earned enough people's attention that eventually they all couldn't fit in such small places. The word spread and more admirers followed and so the owners of the performing hall just around the corner allowed her to dance for just one night!"

Morgan clutched onto the shoes, feeling privileged to be holding garments that were once owned by a relative so inspirational.

"However, they were flooded each night with audiences wanting to see Beatrix the remarkable dancer that they had to keep opening the doors and within her career she earned enough money to buy those beautiful shoes. No lights needed, my dear, just her and the piano."

Morgan's spirits were immediately lifted as the shoes were still fixed to her hands.

She waved as she watched her Grandma and Grandpa get into their car and then she tried the shoes on, which fit her perfectly. Knowing that her Great Grandma had the same condition made her feel content knowing she wasn't alone.

Morgan looked down at the shoes and smiled; she had been filled with such hope.

"There are also special dance classes you can attend, which don't have flashing lights, Morgan!" her mother smiled. Morgan soon remembered the note that was written in the book and nodded with pride. She knew exactly what she would write in her first page of her diary.

'Dancing' Morgan wrote, *'best birthday ever!'*

ATONIC

Jimmy: A tonic? Like water?

Dylan: No, not like water, it's called atonic. Atonic seizure.

Jimmy: What is it? I've never heard of that. A seizure is a seizure, right?

Dylan: Wrong! There are more than 20 different seizure disorders; some that are caused by other conditions; they don't need to be epilepsy. However atonic seizures are just one type of seizure to do with epilepsy and in epilepsy alone there are around 40 known seizures.

Jimmy: So what's atonic then?

Dylan: Well, ATONIC seizures are also known as DROP ATTACKS. Suddenly the person having the seizure loses muscle tone, which can make them fall and seriously hurt themselves.

Jimmy: Ouch. That sounds painful.

Dylan: It is, it usually takes a few seconds up to a minute to recover and regain consciousness; people can seriously injure themselves as well as feel confused or tired!

Jimmy: Just thinking about it hurts my poor head!

Dylan: Exactly, your head is very

important, which is why head gear is available to prevent lumps and bumps when people do have drop attacks, as well as being sensible and avoid using cooking appliances, holding breakable items or walking across the road unassisted.

Jimmy: So who can have atonic seizures then?

Dylan: Absolutely anyone! They are more common in children but occur in all age groups. If you experience this, it is wise to seek medical attention so the doctor can do some tests and see if it is a seizure or something else.

Jimmy: So it can happen to anyone then? There are so many things to fall and trip over- the stairs are an obvious one! Going down the stairs especially is just terrifying!

Dylan: Yes it is, just like anyone, the stairs are a major risk so be careful going up and down them! Especially people who have atonic seizures; I find crawling up the stairs safer and then going down the stairs holding on to the railings and sliding down on your bottom!

Jimmy: That sounds fun.

Dylan: It's certainly safer than falling down them. Image how fun that would be...

Jimmy: It wouldn't be much fun at all.

Dylan: Precisely.

Jimmy: I think I do need a drink after all this information but this time I know the difference between a tonic drink and atonic seizures.

Dylan: Finally…

❖

ALL THE SAME

❖

Your neck or your wrist,

Dog tag? What's this?

Keep calm, don't fret,

It's just a medical bracelet.

Turn it over, just see:

Name, Date, Disability.

Just as long as it's filled out

You're protected with no doubt.

Invisible to the eye,

Strangers walk on by,

Just as long as they've got the name,

You're safe; we're all the same.

CHARLIE'S ONE IN A MILLION!

❖

"Want" Charlie would shout, bouncing up to his bricks in the corner of the room. He adored his coloured bricks with the painted letters on all six sides; the cheery faced boy crossed his legs and sat in front of his box of toys and instantly shovelled them on the floor ready stack them up.

Jenna and Louise were watching him from the open kitchen in Louise's apartment.

"He's attached to them." she

remarked laughing to her sister; they both kept their eyes on the three year old in his stripy blue dungarees as they sipped their cups of coffee.

"Well you're stuck for choices this Christmas then!" Jenna quipped. Charlie was about to start nursery in a week and Louise was anxious about Charlie; he had barely spoken and she was afraid he wouldn't fit in with the other class members.

"Do you reckon he'll be okay?" she bit her lip anxiously, still watching him match the coloured blocks with ease; her eyebrows elevated as she became amazed and completely forgot about her conversation. "Look! Look! Look at what he's done!" she pointed to the stack of blocks and Jenna bobbed her head around the corner to see his impressive masterpiece.

"Yes! See, that right there, that's proof that he will be more than okay!" her sister folded her arms and let out a smug half smile.

Later that day, Charlie lifted his leg rubbing his thigh up against the sofa's front; she peered down and saw he was trying to sit by his mother.

"Aw, Sweetie, why didn't you say that you wanted to sit by Mummy?"

Expecting some sort of gesture from her son, she scooped him up by his underarms and sat him next to her, giving him a cuddle, "How are you my clever little man?"

"Ehr" he blurted, shunning her away; he settled his tongue comfortably above his open bottom lip and let his dribble cast on his cheeks and chin.

She grimaced, pulling her sleeve over her hand, and wiped his face clean. His lack of speech concerned Louise.

"Charlie?" her smile faded as she noticed her son had suddenly become fixated with the television, "Charlie?" she repeated. She hoped the added emphasis would earn his attention but he still wasn't listening. "Charlie!"

She swivelled her son's body around to face her. "Why aren't you paying attention?"

The child let out a shrill scream; he dribbled once more and reverted to the television. Louise's soft touch outweighed her anger and frustration, which would often allow Charlie to behave how he did. She let out a sigh and gently brushed his fringe sideways and once more he let out a scream as she did so.

Louise often felt punished; her reclusive nature resulted from her divorce from her husband when Charlie was just weeks old. Her outlets consisted of her sister's visits and emails from her friend, Denise, who had recently emigrated to Athos.

She felt Charlie's lack of progression was due to being a bad mother; her bookshelf was overridden with books about parenting to ensure she did everything perfectly.

Her nails were in a constant cycle of being bitten down, more so as the week passed, and the day finally arrived where Charlie wore his smart grey polo shirt, which tucked into his best blue joggers.

"It's okay" Louise reassured him bending down outside the nursery gates; Charlie wouldn't stop bawling. His echo of dedicated screaming captured the other parents' attention. Louise tried to hide her embarrassment as more people turned towards the scene.

Eventually Charlie calmed down and trod down the ramp leading to the nursery. A teacher greeted him with a wave but Charlie ignored her kind gesture; finally the string of children disappeared into the building and the door closed.

"I hope he's going to be okay." Louise chuntered to herself as she closed her car door; she turned on the radio hoping it would act as an adequate distraction and closed her eyes.

"Hello?" a woman mouthed as she knocked on the car. Louise shot up and rolled down the window.

"Can I help you?" Louise asked the lady with grey permed hair; she glanced down and saw she was holding a small wicker basket.

"Would you like to help raise money for Down's syndrome?" she asked in a soft, Irish lilt. Louise bit her lip and glanced discreetly at the basket that contained donations.

"I already donate!" she let out an awkward chuckle.

"Sorry to bother you!" the lady replied; she left Louise to wind up the window and walked down the path.

Louise sighed and slumped back into her car seat, reeling up the music once more. She felt slightly guilty for lying to the woman but a charity was something she hadn't ever considered before. She didn't even know what Down's Syndrome was; in fact, she hardly knew anything about disabilities as no one in her family had a condition as far as she was aware.

Louise finally drove off the school's premises and returned home; as the front door to her apartment burst open she made a beeline for the sofa and drifted off to sleep.

Moments later she received a phone call which disrupted her nap; it was her sister.

"Oh, it's you." she gruffly sounded, rubbing her eyes.

"Cheers! Nice to hear your voice too!" came a satirical reply, "I just phoned to see how you got on. Was it emotional?"

"Don't start." Louise's voice seemed monotonous; her lack of enthusiasm and light-heartedness was suppressed by complete upset, "I just miss him and hope he's coping well."

"Louise, he'll be fine!" Jenna sighed; Louise was oblivious to being a clingy mother but her sister could see it and thought comfort was something she needed right now, "I'll come over-it's my day off."

Louise put the phone down as the conversation ended and she resumed to her original position on the sofa. Once Jenna had arrived she noticed that Louise had turned eyeballing the clock into an obsession, calculating the hours left for picking up Charlie from school, and soon enough the time came.

"It's time to pick up Charlie!" she jumped up, leaving her half empty cup on the side table. "Are you coming?"

Jenna stared in horror at her hysterical sister and grabbed her handbag as they headed towards the car. "Jeez, why do you need the music that loud?" Jenna grimaced as the radio came on. She could see her sister wasn't interested in sisterly criticism and so she conjured up reassuring words instead, "Charlie's first day will have gone well." she said, studying her anomalous behaviour.

"I hope so." Louise replied. As they reached the school, a row of parents were patiently waiting for their children to exit the building; the door swung open and excited faces painted on children ran out to their family members, jumping up to give them a welcoming hug. Well, all except for one child: Charlie. He eventually plodded out of the building clutching onto his favourite action figure.

"Why hasn't he got a friend?" Louise fretted, "Why isn't he as happy as all the other children?"

"I don't know, Louise, maybe he's tired?"

"He doesn't look tired. He's never tired. He always sleeps well!" she was suddenly interrupted by Jenna's impatient response.

"He has had a busy day, Louise, he is probably tired! Just relax."

Charlie finally met his Aunt Jenna and mother. Louise bent down, seeming emotionally unsteady, and hugged her precious son; he stood there rigidly gawking at the surroundings.

"Did you enjoy today?" she hesitated, stroking his blonde hair. Charlie hated his mother touching his hair and so he moved and placed his action figure in his mouth before plodding towards the car.

The evening flew by and Jenna decided to return home; she could see Louise's eyes were miserable and dull.

"If you need me, you know where I am." she gave Louise a hug and waved to Charlie before she left. Charlie was playing with his building blocks, neatly piling them into the same scheme, and as Louise glanced at the time she pouted; she had not yet spoken with her son about his big day.

"Time for bed!" she began tidying the blocks off the floor blocking out Charlie's horrendous screaming and lashing out as she piled them up into the red toy box.

After a tiring hour Charlie soon went to bed and slept.

"*I can do this.*" she whispered to herself whilst watching over him.

As the days emerged together Louise's behaviour improved as her son came back every day without a qualm.

"Have you had a lovely day?" she asked. Charlie looked up; a girl with strawberry blonde pigtails skipped by and waved to Charlie, "Bye, Charlie!" she exclaimed. Charlie had no desire to reciprocate and ignored her.

"Say goodbye, Charlie!" Louise goaded; shocked at his ignorance. She waved to the girl on his behalf before they headed home.

A month swiftly flew by when Louise received an unexpected phone call from Charlie's school.

"Hello this is Charlie's teacher, Mrs Fortridge. I would like to meet with Charlie's mother." Louise clasped onto the phone.

"Sure. It isn't serious is it?" she started chewing her nails as she awaited the teacher's response.

"I just would like to discuss a few things with you, Miss Smith."

"When would be the best time to come to down?" Louise asked; her heart drummed out of her chest as she listened intently.

"Would today after school be convenient?" Louise scribbled the important information on her notepad.

"Yes. Thank you." she replied. After the phone call Louise sat down thinking about all the worst possibilities, "What if he's been injured or bullied?" she uttered recalling back to his quiet behaviour in the playground. "Maybe that's why he hasn't spoken to anyone!"

The hands on the clock teased the unsettled mother until it was time for her to leave the apartment; she bolted out of the room and slammed the door.

"For crying out loud!" she gritted her teeth as she caught her finger in the door. The encore of panic clouded her vision, "I've got a pounding headache!" she mumbled. She unclenched her teeth and fumbled for her car keys. The stress that had been building up for years made her feel numb but she was in denial of her illness and so she continued to suffer in silence with constant numbness and head pains.

The parents had formed a group of

friends at their children's nursery. Louise, being her solitary self, hadn't yet found the courage to speak with anyone; she had her usual routine of standing up the corner waiting for her son to exit the school.

Again the line of children snaked in the direction of their parents. Anxiously, Louise waited for people to disperse before taking Charlie's hand and making her way up to the reception area.

"I'm here to see Charlie's teacher." Louise forced a smile to the dark haired receptionist.

"Come through." she replied monotonously. A lady with short

bobbed hair briskly walked towards Louise and Charlie. She held out her hand.

"Hi there, I'm Mrs Fortridge, pleased to meet you." her face had a welcoming smile. "Follow me and we will have a little chat."

They sat down in an empty classroom and Charlie sat cross-legged on the floor finding some building blocks to play with.

"What is Charlie like at home, Mrs Smith?"

"Miss-" Louise corrected her. "He is happy. He likes being at home and on weekends we go to the local park; it's usually really early because he doesn't like to go when the other children are there." she chuckled nervously. The teacher nodded as she placed her finger over her lips.

"Do you speak about school with him?" she asked, crossing her legs; Louise slanted her head to the side quizzically. Her mouth became a little dry as her nerves revisited once more, which made her hesitate.

"I try but he seems a little reluctant to discuss things with me. Why are you asking me these questions, Mrs Fortridge?" her defensive nature struck and so the teacher calmly placed her notepad on the desk, which contained the useful information.

"Charlie has been expressing behaviour, which I believe have some traits of a condition called Autism. As he is only three years old, we cannot tell as all children his age can express the symptoms yet not have it. However, I have noticed Charlie over the past weeks and I am concerned, which is why I have arranged this meeting with you."

Louise's eyes grew in shock. "I can't believe it! What exactly has he been doing?"

"I have noticed his lack of communication with the other pupils and his frequent aggressive behaviour; he is happy to share his lunch, yet other things, such as toys, he screams and sometimes hits out." Louise froze. She couldn't believe what she was hearing as this wasn't the same little boy she was taking home every day at three o'clock.

"His language is a little delayed." Louise admitted, "I am aware of that."

She decided not to disclose stories about Charlie's outbursts.

"Miss Smith, perhaps it would be a good idea to seek your personal doctor." she advised, "Each case of autism is different and unique to the child so a more thorough investigation could help."

As their meeting adjourned, they

stood up and exchanged handshakes.

"Thank you, Mrs Fortridge" she said straining a smile, "I will book an appointment with the doctor first thing tomorrow!" Louise looked down at her son, who was sat playing with the building blocks; she closed her eyes for a minute and recalled the conversation with her sister in her apartment. *"He'll be more than okay!"*

"Is that why he's doing that all the time?" Louise pointed towards the array of synchronised blocks.

"It can be a trait." the teacher concurred, "But like I said, it can just be fine. It's best to find out." she smiled, "I hope everything goes well for you tomorrow."

As Louise drove home with her son, tears threatened to break from her eyes. Denial was her immediate mechanism she used to block out difficult situations but this particular subject was harder to ignore.

Later that night Louise lay in bed, reiterating the teacher's words in her head, whilst uncontrollably sobbing; she stared at her alarm clock until it finally sounded out at seven o'clock.

Her son was already awake, waiting to get dressed for school.

"We're not going to nursery today, sweetheart." Louise softly spoke as she slipped his clothes on him. "We are going to see the doctor instead."

Louise dashed about the apartment before heading out the door with her son. She was so anxious about his appointment.

They found themselves waiting in the doctor's surgery; the room where they sat made the place seem promising with the number of brightly painted walls and the modern play area, situated in the corner, welcome to all children.

Soon appeared Jenna, panting whilst tucking her car keys in her jean pocket; she waited a moment to compose herself and sat down beside her sister. She ruffled Charlie's hair, disregarding his reserved preference, and turned towards Louise.

"Goodness, you look rough." she remarked, studying the dark lines under her eyes. "Could you not sleep?"

Louise raised her eyebrows at Jenna and shook her head. "I'm glad you could make it" Louise replied. Her exhausted disposition toyed with her emotions and her battle with holding back tears seemed almost impossible.

They waited patiently in the quiet room, listening to the loud crunching of the clock as it calculated the minutes, until a door opened.

"Charles Smith" the doctor called; the three stood up in a synchronised manner and headed into the room. As the tall doctor plummeted into his chair he scooped his pen and a pad together whilst letting out a warm compelling smile. He quickly assessed him before nodding.

"I'm going to refer him to a specific kind of doctor." he said, clicking away on the computer, "It will take a few weeks but he specialises in disorders and will be able to do various tests to make the right diagnoses."

Jenna and Louise looked towards one another. They felt sick but all they could do was wait.

The inevitable day came where Charlie had to visit the specific doctor at the hospital, and as promised, Jenna accompanied her sister and Charlie for moral support. As they approached the room, a man stood in the doorway.

"Hello there I'm Doctor Davison, a Paediatrician psychiatrist." He greeted. His bald oval-shaped head accompanied by an oversized beard gave him a friendly façade. Louise bunched her hands in the sleeves of her cardigan; his constant need to click his mouse made Louise even more nervous as she took is as a bad sign.

Suddenly he stopped at stared at the computer screen, reading a small paragraph before returning to their discussion.

"So, you say Charles has developed a noticeable pattern in his behaviour which has concerned you?" he queried. Louise nodded erratically. Her lips had a slight redness about them from biting them frequently.

The doctor studied the small boy sitting on a small chair, dangling his legs, and placed his hand on his beard.

"Okay then, Charles." he stood up and walked towards the other side of the room, "Come with me."

Charlie dismissed his request and stared at the posters that were dotted about on the walls.

"Charlie!" Louise whispered sharply, "Go towards the nice man please." he continued gawping at the posters; Louise turned an intense shade of red due to embarrassment.

"It's okay." the doctor reassured, "Does he normally ignore you like this? If you say his name, does he seem to listen to you or is he more likely to ignore you?"

Humiliated, Louise took a deep breath and started. Jenna was only aware of a few things but Louise felt as though confessing her difficulty would make her sound like an inept mother.

"He doesn't really listen to me. I do talk to Charlie but it's as though he's constantly distracted by other things."

Doctor Davison turned towards Charlie and called his name again, putting more emphasis than he did previously.

"Charlie!" he corrected; he wondered whether using his nickname would have a different outcome but it didn't.

Louise's face paraded a horrified expression as she witnessed the problem; she knew Doctor Davison's frequent scribbling on his notepad wasn't a good sign.

"I've noticed he doesn't make eye contact either, Miss Smith." He started clicking his fingers near to Charlie's left ear subsequently following his right, "He isn't deaf." he added as Charlie reacted to the loud noise.

"I took him to the doctors months ago and they concluded his hearing was perfect, which is why I presumed he was just being ignorant or unfocused!" she let out a nervous laugh as she watched him scribble on his pad once more.

Louise justified Charlie's excessive screaming as the doctor snapped his fingers once more by Charlie's ears.

"I've noticed that he's very sensitive to noise, such as: the hairdryer, hoover, cake whisker, motorbikes..." her list trailed off as he wrote down on his pad again.

Charlie moved towards a low yellow table that sat in the corner of the room and perched on the chair that faced it; he immediately snatched the blue plastic box and pulled out some toys.

He made no eye contact with the ladies as he read out some questions on his documents; Jenna and Louise knew these questions would help confirm a diagnosis for Charlie and so the women sat up in their seats and placed their hands in their laps.

"Is Charlie getting on at school okay?"

"Yes" Louise squeaked.

"I bet he has lots of friends." he

looked up and smiled at Louise, who now looked agitated.

"He does." she peered over his shoulder watching him reiterate her words into a sprawled mess on paper; her humiliation caused her to bend the truth.

"You told me he has no friends!" Jenna whispered; the doctor sat back and waited for the statement to elaborate.

"I didn't mean literally!" Louise turned towards her sister hastily exchanging a stony glare. She huffed and turned towards Doctor Davison.

"His nursery teacher noticed he hadn't the best communication skills. I haven't seen him with any classmates; In fact he is always the last one out and alone. However he wakes up and is eager to go to nursery every morning!"

"I see. Well do you know whether Charles expresses aggression towards others?" he queried.

"No." she lied, feeling shameful.

"Yes he does!" Jenna corrected, "He doesn't like his hair being touched!" she nudged her chair forward and spoke directly to the doctor.

"He loves playing with his toys but if you try and play with him and touch them- all hell is let loose!" she turned towards her sister, "He is asking these questions to help Charlie and to help you too; he only needs to know this information to diagnose him correctly; he's not going to judge you, Louise."

Louise looked to the floor and realised Jenna was right.

"His teacher has noticed frequent outbursts. She spoke with me and mentioned Charlie can be very possessive of his toys and violent if others try and play with them." he put his pen to the paper and nodded.

Louise watched her son bashing the toys into one another, giggling and enjoying himself; she smiled, seeing how content he was in his own little world, and then turned to the doctor completely oblivious to the next question.

"How close are you and Charles? Does he hug you?"

"Very rarely." she shook her head, recalling the last memory she had of them, snuggled up on the sofa in front of the television, yet the solitary memory had slipped away making her feel unfulfilled, "I'm a single mother. I feel our relationship has grown apart ever since his father and I split up."

His fingers slotted together as he pushed back into his chair; he watched her eyebrows turn in and tears started to appear.

"Charlie ignores me, he bites, he

screams, he kicks, he's left bruises and marks, I can't guess what he wants at times- I ask him but he won't tell me!"

She closed her eyes and let the tears roll down her cheeks. She took a deep breath and turned towards her child, "But he's Charlie and I love him."

Charlie stood still, looking out the window, indifferently; he watched the birds swirling in the sky making wonderful shapes.

Jenna placed her arm around Louise's shoulder; the doctor paused and decided it was time to speak about the confirmed diagnoses.

"It's autism isn't it?" Louise stared

in horror. The Doctor Davison aided the lady with a box of tissues.

"There is no cure for autism, Miss Smith. However there are certain therapies that can bring about substantial improvement, and of course there's family counselling." the words were becoming more fluent, making her less distraught, inevitably reassuring her.

"That's perfect." Jenna smiled. She turned towards Louise, who let out a relieved laugh.

"Also medication may be prescribed if ever he displays anything such as: depression, anxiety, OCD."

"I've heard of dietary plans as

well!" Jenna chimed in, excusing her enthusiastic outburst.

"Yes, they do." he nodded, "Very rarely but it's another suggestion."

Louise wiped the remaining tears from her eyes; suddenly she didn't feel alone and felt comforted by the amount of choices.

"Thank you." she stood up and gratefully shook the doctor's hand. Charlie bolted out of the door and so the three headed out the door.

"How do you feel?" Jenna turned to her sister once they arrived back at Louise's apartment. Louise didn't hesitate to show how relieved she was and smiled.

"I am so happy, Jen, who knew there were so many different possibilities for Charlie?"

Evening passed and Jenna was ready to go home.

"It's been a long day." she hugged Louise, "But at least we now know the right path for Charlie and he can be a happier child now we understand." she slung her handbag over her shoulder and waved to Charlie before leaving the apartment.

Louise parachuted on the settee and turned on the television, making sure her son was content enough with his toys; she then began thinking about the busy day they'd had.

"It's going to be fine, Charlie!" she smiled; she was aware that her son's behaviour wasn't going to change immediately but she felt as though she had a new insight to things. She thought back to the doctor's remark,

"People with autism respond well to routine; they simply thrive off it."

"That makes so much sense. He's always up extremely early ready for nursery." she whispered out loud.

Charlie stopped playing with his toys and galloped over to the sofa, where Louise was comfortably slouching; she tucked her hands under his arms and positioned him next to her.

"There's about one in a hundred people in the UK like you!" she said to her son, remembering the statistics from the doctor. Charlie stared at the television, only this time Louise understood and she smiled, "But you, Charlie, are one in a million!"

AN INSIDE GENIUS

Singer and guitarist,

James Durbin.

English naturalist,

Charles Darwin.

American cartoonist,

Charles M. Schulz.

Rockstar,

Craig Nicholls.

Director and writer,

Woody Allen.

Systems administrator,

Gary McKinnon.

King of Pop,

Michael Jackson,

TV Puppeteer,

James Henson.

Third president of America,

Thomas Jefferson.

Light-bulb inventor,

Thomas Edison.

Renaissance painter,

Michelangelo (di Lodovico Buonarotti

Simoni).

Pokémon creator,

Satoshi Tajiri.

Theoretical physicist,

Einstein.

American author,

Mark Twain.

Composer and pianist,

Ludwig Van Beethoven,

Author and poet,

Hans Christian Andersen.

Film director and producer,

Sir Alfred Hitchcock, KBE.

Scottish painter,

Peter Howson, OBE.

Natural philosopher and scientist,

Henry Cavendish.

Fashion model,

Heather Kuzmich.

Business magnate and philanthropist,

Bill Gates, KBE.

Presenter, comedian and writer,

Michael Palin, CBE.

British author,

Luke Jackson.

Greatest English scientist,

Isaac Newton.

British novelist,

Jane Austen.

Elecro-Pop Pioneer,

Gary Newman.

Novelist,

George Orwell,

Classical composer,

Mozart.

All with Asperger's syndrome;

Genius.

X AND Y

Jimmy: Who is Doctor Langdon Down?

Dylan: Have you ever heard of Down's Syndrome?

Jimmy: No. What is that?

Dylan: It is a genetic condition where a person inherits an extra chromosome.

Jimmy: Wait… What's a chromosome?

Dylan: A chromosome is a thread-like structure that carries thousands of hereditary genes. Genes are what gives us our physical traits, such as eye and hair colour that get passed on from our mother and father.

Jimmy: I see. How many chromosomes do we have?

Dylan: forty-six. However, people with Down's Syndrome have an extra chromosome!

Jimmy: Forty-seven chromosomes…

Dylan: That's correct. The likelihood of having a baby born with Down's Syndrome increases with age.

Jimmy: So, who is Doctor Langdon Down?

Dylan: He's who Down's Syndrome is named after. Doctor Langdon Down was the person who first described

Down's Syndrome in 1866!

Jimmy: That's a long time ago. How common is Down's Syndrome?

Dylan: Seven hundred and fifty babies are born with it in the UK per year; it affects all races and religions and it's one of the most common genetic birth defects.

Jimmy: What are the defects?

Dylan: There are a few things which affect the person. It can affect their physical appearance as well as their health.

Jimmy: What physical traits can people with Down's Syndrome have?

Dylan: Typical physical traits include: flat facial features, hypermobility, where the person has the ability to extend their joints, an enlarged tongue, upwards slant on the eyes, short stature and low muscle tone.

Jimmy: That is a lot.

Dylan: Yes. There are lots more characteristics though; normally babies with Down's Syndrome appear 'floppy' due to low muscle tone.

Jimmy: How about health risks?

Dylan: Complications can include: learning difficulties, heart disorders, infections, thyroid dysfunctions, cervical spine dislocation, blood disorders, hearing and vision impairments, gastrointestinal issues, muscle tone and growth.

Jimmy: Is there a cure for Down's Syndrome?

Dylan: No but there's plenty of support groups that can improve the person's lifestyle and check-ups with healthcare specialists to provide help.

Jimmy: Like?

Dylan: Like physiotherapists, dieticians and speech therapists.

Jimmy: That's encouraging!

Dylan: It is.

Jimmy: Speaking of genes, I need to go shopping to buy some new ones!

GREGG AND ME

❖

I sat there in front of the interviewer and placed my glass of cool water onto the desk. The silence filled the room and my nerves got the better of me, making my thumbs rotate around one another as my hands clasped together.

"So, Edward, please tell me about yourself." the interviewer smiled. As she sat on the edge of the suite in her pinstripe skirt and white blouse the most apparent thing about her were the smudges of lipstick on her front tooth.

"Err…I'm Edward Carter and I'm twenty three years old. I live in Bristol and-"

Immediately I was interrupted. The interviewer was taken aback as he was so rude to disrupt me.

"I live in Bristol" the second voice said in a quieter tone, "I live in Bristol."

Both of us overrode the situation as it was my interview, and so we continued.

"I play sports" I snorted, "I enjoy tennis because it takes my mind off things." I snorted again; it was the middle of November and the bitter weather was desperate to invite itself in the warm heated room where they were seated; I snorted for the third time as I reached for the glass of water.

"No." the other voice uttered and pinched me; the interviewer looked stunned and began writing in her notepad. This behaviour was quite extraordinary and something she wasn't use to.

"Are you okay Edward?" she asked, "Do you want to stop?"

"No, it's alright. It's Gregg, he can be like that." I chuckled slightly, slightly embarrassed at his behaviour. However, I continued, "Tennis has helped me relax, everything is the same in my life, but tennis makes things more manageable I guess!" I smiled and took the glass of water off the table without any disruption.

I answered more questions and spoke as best as I could about my favourite hobbies, interests and personal details for my words to be published in the following month's magazine.

"You are a very influential icon, Edward" the interviewer smiled, showing her gleaming teeth, marked with her pink lipstick.

"Thanks." I bashfully grinned, looking down at the floor, covering half of my face in my grey polo top.

As the interviewer dictated my

words onto the clipboard that rested on her knee she found herself more comfortable around Gregg as his outbursts of disruptions were less aggressive and carried on writing her summary of the half hour interview; as he giggled, clapped and yelped, the interviewer got accustomed to him.

That half hour made her see how easy it was for me to look after Gregg; although sometimes it was difficult and harmful, but it was acceptable.

"It was nice meeting you, Edward!" the interviewer shook my hand, "And I'm glad you have such a positive outlook on having Tourette's syndrome"

"I call it 'Gregg' because it makes the situation less serious." I replied, shaking her hand. Before she exited the building I sat back and added "It was a pleasure meeting you too."

❖

AM I STILL YOUR HERO?

❖

I was six foot two and everyone knew

me as a cheeky, handsome man.

"I am a soldier" is how I'd introduce

myself, "I'll be fighting in

Afghanistan."

I took a picture for my family,

"Remember my face before my duty,

For these scars I will endure so

remember me by beauty;

My blonde hair will soon be lost and

my boyish grin will fade,

My thoughts will start turning sour;

my smile's willpower will soon
degrade."
I was a muscular man, with strong
arms and legs, trained for this mission,
Envious friends, proud daughter and
loving wife; this is for Afghan's
commission.
'Dear mom' is what every letter starts
with; strong headed but soft hearted,
I try to escape by closing my eyes as
another dead body is departed.
I am alert and my heart pounds hard;
in a team we commit.
"Man down" is that destroying word,
yet we never will quit.
That man was me; I fell to the floor so
numb,

Muffled screams blare out to my
heart's arrhythmic drum.
I was fortunate that only my legs were
discarded from myself,
I was sent back home, reunited with
my family, along with everybody else.
Physically different but I'm still the
same, the one that's fought for this
land,
It doesn't matter what size, I have
dignity and pride; I'm more than a
cheeky, handsome man.

SIMPLE OR COMPLEX?

❖

Jimmy: I've been hearing about Tourette's Syndrome. It is so confusing!

Dylan: Which bit, the Simple or Complex part?

Jimmy: I wouldn't say it was simple…

Dylan: No. There are two categories, there are involuntary movements with Tourette's syndrome called tics, and they are either Simple or Complex.

Jimmy: Oh! I understand now- so

what's the difference then?

Dylan: With Simple, you get tic movements which may include: vocal tics, such as yelping or shouting, snorting or sniffing and other varied noises or more physical tics, such as eye rolling, eye blinking or lip smacking.

Jimmy: Oh, I see- that explains it better now. However, it still doesn't sound very simple! How about complex tics?

Dylan: Well, just like the Simple tics, Complex tics are also involuntary. They may have traits of: punching and hitting out, body jerking, humming or whistling, yelling or stuttering.

Jimmy: That is a lot!

Dylan: There are so much more; those are just some. Some even include coprolalia and copopraxia.

Jimmy: What is that?

Dylan: Well, coprolalia is an utterance of obscene, derogatory or socially inappropriate words and copopraxia is making obscene gestures.

Jimmy: Is this typical of Tourette's Syndrome?

Dylan: People associate Tourette's Syndrome with swearing but that is a stereotype; in fact only a small percentage of people display these.

Jimmy: I wonder what triggers a tic.

Dylan: Tics can fluctuate. However,

they may be more frequent with stress and anxiety and if you're feeling under the weather with illnesses such as infections. As well as being frequent, they could be more intense.

Jimmy: Yikes! Who can have Tourette's Syndrome then?

Dylan: Anyone! It is an inherited neurological disorder and although Tourette's Syndrome can occur at any age, it generally appears before the age of eighteen, it is usually noticed in very early childhood.

Jimmy: Is there anything that can help?

Dylan: Definitely, there's medication that can help. Medication such as antihypertensives, used for controlling high blood pressure, muscle relaxants for when muscles become too stiff, and neuroleptics, which blocks the effects of dopamine in the brain.

Jimmy: That is great!

Dylan: It is, medication that suits the patient will help as best as possible, and this way people with the syndrome will be able to enjoy the benefits of sports, leisure or fun hobbies, such as cooking!

Jimmy: You've just reminded me...I've left the oven on!

THE HURDLES

The doctor explains the rules, "You have multiple sclerosis" he diagnoses; the patient sits down, ready in position, and the room's silence spreads for a moment.

They anxiously wait for the loud bang of the hospital's documents, ready to be placed on the desk.

The patient's adrenaline rushes, her heart races, whilst the roar of the doctor speaks; the hurdles she will face throughout life could alternate. She understands that sometimes she would be able to race, sometimes she wouldn't; but she was determined to think about the hurdles she could jump, being positive and strong, being a winner.

The arena is empty; the only people present are the doctor, who is speaking in solace, and the patient burying her head in her hands; she is preparing for the event, awaiting the supporter's response.

At the end of the meeting the doctor hands over the documents; she grips it with both hands and suddenly her eyes line with tears. The overwhelming atmosphere draws to a close; she shakes the doctor's hand as she receives her notes and graciously leaves the room, taking a deep breath, holding in the abundance of emotions.

She returns home and sits in front of her husband. As he interviews her, curious about her news, she speaks,

"I have been diagnosed with multiple sclerosis."

Her husband sits closer, creating more of an intimate space, and she starts reiterating the devastating news.

"What is multiple sclerosis?" he questions suddenly, waiting patiently for her next words.

"It's a progressive neurological disease. It damages the sheathes of the nerve cells in the brain and spinal cord."

He nods, "…and how are you feeling?"

She lets out a smile yet her eyes look dim. Her world crumbles around her as she feels exhausted; regardless of the amount of support, she feels alone.

"Horrible." she replies. "There are too many obstacles!"

They speak about the present and the future, the ups and the downs, and once they come to an understanding she regains her happy, confident self; prepared to face the hurdles once more.

MY GRANDDAD

I was only three when my granddad passed away. I'm not implying I have an immaculate memory but I often marvel how my ability of remembering so far back.

I am now twenty-two, which will give some concept of how long ago this was. The chair still sits opposite the television in my living room where he used to sit; it was renowned as 'Granddad's chair' as he would always sit there. He sat in his chair with my brother and I standing either side; we were giggling hysterically as he continued to turn around in his chair to tickle us. We would hide behind the chair and eventually appear over and over again; he always brought a smile to our faces with his daftness.

The fondest memory I have is where I feel content and utterly loved; I was sat on my granddad's knee, wearing my pink pyjamas and I watched the television as my mum, nan and granddad happily conversed. I thought he was one of the tallest and strongest people in the world; little did I know he was classed as 'average height' and had a disability.

It wasn't until a few years ago that I learnt that my granddad had a few health complications; he suffered a stroke at an early age along with a series of unfortunate struggles that compromised his health. His life was prematurely and unfairly taken.

From a young age you are conditioned to see things through rose-tinted glasses but as you learn more and get older, deception unfortunately pollutes them.

I didn't ever contemplate the number of walking sticks that were propped up the one corner of my grandparent's house; in fact I just took it for granted as grandparents were supposed to have that 'old' stereotype with permed hair with a walking stick, rounded glasses and the obsession to knit away in front of the fire.

I was amazed to discover his incredible talent of playing the organ and piano. My nan mentioned 'Moonlight Sonata' was one of his favourite pieces; a beautiful piece albeit a tricky composition.

A story about his difficulty finding the right words frustrated me as some people are so ignorant, unaware of the annoyance it causes stroke victims; as I've gotten older I have encountered people who have suffered strokes and have seen how mentally and physically debilitating it is for them, not to mention life-changing. Keeping a positive outlook is a difficult yet excellent method to recovery and I'd like to think my granddad did so; judging from the photographs I've seen I reckon he did.

Many people are ignorant of the disability, some can be kind and helpful, some conscious, some insecure and others can just be undeniably rude; I personally put that down to their lack knowledge and fear of something they don't understand.

Not only did my granddad play the organ and piano, he played football for one of the best football teams of his time; he featured on a newspaper along with his team members on the front page.

If a toddler of three years could see past a person's disability, I am confident an adult would have ten times the ability to do the same. Illnesses don't control you, you control them; I know as I've seen solid proof and I can honestly say he is an inspiration and the reason why I like to see the brighter side to my own ailments.

My amazing Granddad Walter (August 25 1933 – June 2 1994.)

CVA AND TIA

Jimmy: What are you doing?

Dylan: *reading leaflet* Looking at some facts on strokes.

Jimmy: Why?

Dylan: Because it wouldn't hurt to do some research. I have found out some interesting facts. Have you ever heard of a 'cerebrovascular accident'?

Jimmy: No.

Dylan: How about a 'transient ischemic attack'?

Jimmy: No.

Dylan: Well, these are two types of stroke.

Jimmy: Firstly, what is a stroke?

Dylan: A stroke is an attack to the brain; your brain needs constant blood supply for it to function, which provides important nutrients and oxygen to the brain cells in order to keep them alive. However, when a person has a stroke, it cuts off the blood supply to part of the brain and brain cells are damaged!

Jimmy: Could the brain cells die?

Dylan: Yes. Now you know what a stroke is you can learn about the differences.

Jimmy: Oh no, not big words again!

Dylan: Relax! Firstly a cerebrovascular accident is what we have just spoken about, but there are so many more things to look out for when someone is having one.

Jimmy: Like what?

Dylan: Well, like signs to look out for and what to do if someone is having a stroke.

Jimmy: Oh no, I wouldn't know what to do!

Dylan: Exactly my point. There are some key points to watch out for when someone is having a stroke; they are very distinct because they happen so quickly. These include: trouble seeing, slurred speech, weakness on one side and difficulty walking.

Jimmy: What could someone do to help?

Dylan: Simply phone an ambulance. The emergency services will take them to hospital and the sooner they act the better! In the meantime, ask them to repeat an easy sentence and check if their speech is slurred. You could also ask the person to bob their tongue out to see if their mouth is lop-sided.

Jimmy: What else could I do?

Dylan: You could ask them if they could raise both arms. Typically it is the left arm that is weaker so if you notice one arm isn't raised as high as the other, that's another indication.

Jimmy: Will they get better?

Dylan: About a third of stroke patients have a significant recovery in just a month! However, that's not the case for everyone; most have long-term problems and it may take up to a year, maybe a little longer, for the best recovery.

Jimmy: That sounds like a lot of hard work and very frustrating for them.

Dylan: I am sure it is. Now you have learned about cerebrovascular accidents, how about we learn about Transient Ischemic Attacks (TIAs)...

Jimmy: Are they the same as they're both types of stroke?

Dylan: No. A cerebrovascular accident

is a cut off from the blood supply in the brain whereas a transient ischemic attack is caused by a temporary fall in the blood supply to part of the brain; this leads to lack of oxygen to the brain.

Jimmy: Ah! Why do these happen?

Dylan: If you have high cholesterol and high blood pressure you are putting yourself at risk, not only for a transient ischemic attack but for a cerebrovascular accident as well. They can also cause heart attacks!

Jimmy: I may want to watch what I drink and eat in future.

Dylan: Sometimes it doesn't have to be your lifestyle, it can be hereditary;

if your father or even his father had high cholesterol or high blood pressure, I wouldn't be too surprised if you had it as well!

Jimmy: Well I think I know quite a bit on CVA and TIA now… Time for some TLC!

PICASSO SO HELPFUL

Olivia unravelled her dark hair and let it drape onto her shoulder once more before plaiting it; as she sat quietly at the back of the coach she observed the unruly teenagers pummel the back of the chairs and flick scrunched up pieces of paper at one another. She peered out of the window, hoping to drown out the infantile behaviour for the remaining journey.

The teacher stood up as the vehicle eventually stopped and announced,

"Form a fashionable line." the masculine woman wore a grey suit; she was intimidating with a harsh appearance to match. Her belligerence was enough to question her profession.

Olivia stood up and placed her bag over her shoulder. She waited for the queue to disperse before exiting; Olivia was a renowned loner and isolated herself from the rest as she preferred her own company.

"Make useful and informative notes on what you see today and we shall meet back here at four o'clock."

Everyone held notepads and pens in their hands, "And behave yourselves!" she added before they were dismissed.

Olivia watched everyone head off in various directions as she dawdled behind, sensing the teacher only a couple of feet behind her. Her eyes grew wider; she didn't want to end up conversing with Mrs Madworth, or even worse, having her as company.

"Olivia!" came a cackle. Olivia froze with fear in a muddy puddle; the teacher caught up with her.

"I've noticed you haven't got a partner!"

"I didn't want one!" she squeaked, avoiding eye contact.

"Don't be like that!" a smile almost cracked through her stony looking face, "I'll accompany you."

Mrs. Madworth was usually a stringent woman but the art excursion made her slightly pleasant as it allowed her to escape from the stress of the mundane work that lay on her desk at the school.

Olivia was a brilliant artist and was exceptionally creative; she would have been more enthusiastic about the trip if it wasn't for Mrs. Madworth overshadowing her.

As they meandered down the footpath, Olivia smiled as she saw a muddy track that lay ahead of a small wooden hut.

"That looks interesting!" Olivia

said, pointing in front. Knowing Mrs. Madworth had a phobia of worms, the girl watched her teacher's face crumble into shock. "Shall we have a look?"

"I don't think I will." she replied shaking her head, "Go ahead and I shall see you at four o'clock."

Curious to what was inside, she peered around the corner; bark lay on the floor and straw seats encircled the dark room making it look somewhat tribal.

Being empty and silent was ideal for Olivia; she crept in in the hut and placed her bag besides her, producing a book. The place had a damp musty smell which repulsed her.

"May I sit with you?" a shadow lingered in the entrance; Olivia tore herself away from the page and squinted upwards.

Awkwardness filled the room as a slender boy walked in and slumped down on the seat adjacent to Olivia.

"What're you reading?" the intruder asked.

"The Catcher in the Rye." Olivia replied bluntly. The boy appearance was extremely pale; he had long brown hair that draped over his face and it hid a good portion of his features, which made him look quite secretive.

"My name's Jake." he interrupted

again. Olivia glanced up at the boy.

"Olivia." she replied unimpressed. He extended his legs outwards as he slouched, allowing the bark to pile up in the centre on the hut; Olivia sighed.

"Why are you here?" he asked. Olivia took a deep sigh and closed her book in frustration. As she looked up she noticed something curious about Jake's appearance.

"None of your business!" she scowled. Her eyes wandered down to his hands and revealed a look of surprise; immediately Jake jolted his arms back and pulled his sleeves over his hands to cover them.

"Sorry. I didn't mean to-" Olivia

sheepishly muttered.

"Well it's rude to stare." his appearance caused him to be defensive and insecure; he sighed realising his reaction was a little hasty and apologised.

"I get a little embarrassed, that's all."

They exchanged a smile; Olivia realised Jake wasn't so bad and his timid nature was the result of his long hair.

"If you don't mind me asking, what is it?" Olivia asked, watching Jake unravel his hands from his sleeves, "Did you burn yourself?"

"No." he replied, "I have lupus."

"Lupus?" she tilted her head "What's that?"

"Basically my immune system isn't too great. It's an autoimmune disease." He remained facing the floor which made it difficult to see his features.

Subtly glancing at his hands, she saw his skin was covered with red blotchy sores. "Is it painful?" she asked.

"Yeah." he nodded casually. "I'm used to it though." He peered at Olivia in the corner of his eye and saw the girl was shaken. "Just the joint pain and swelling gets a little painful."

Olivia soon became oblivious to Jake's sores and as they spoke more,

Jake felt comfortable around Olivia. In fact, he tucked his hair behind his ear, which exposed his face.

"This is my 'Butterfly' rash." he mentioned, pointing to his face.

"Butterfly rash?" she paraphrased, "Why is it called that?

Jake pointed to the affected area on his cheeks and the bridge of his nose.

"The rash sort of looks like a butterfly, don't you think?" his face was red and made up of sores, looking equally painful as his hands.

Olivia smiled; she thought it was an endearing and appropriate name for the markings, "I suppose it does. That's kinda cool!"

Jake looked down and bashfully let out a laugh. He had never had his butterfly rash referred to as cool before and suddenly he found himself feeling a little less insecure about his appearance. The sun immediately beamed through the entrance and through the roof, making it light.

Olivia stood up, "Let's take a walk!" she suggested. Jake seemed reluctant and pulled a face, "Come on! It will be fun!" Olivia persuaded; she grabbed his hand and Jake sluggishly followed.

"So why are you here?" Olivia asked.

"I like to appreciate the art. I live

near here and it's a place that I find comforting and peaceful.

Are you going to tell me why you're here?"

Olivia glowered at the adolescences in the distance, "I'm on an art trip with those reprobates over there."

"I take it you don't like them?" Jake commented. Olivia shook her head.

"Nope." she sounded fragile, "They dismiss me or they bully me; it depends on what mood they're feeling in but it's on a daily basis. I'm just glad I can be away from them for a while."

"You shouldn't hide because of

bullies." Jake said. He realised his words were somewhat hypocritical as that was what he spent most of his life doing.

As they wandered around the gallery they stopped at one particular painting.

"Picasso!" Jake marvelled. "I love this picture!" his eyes glinted as he stood there appreciating the work of art. However, a group of Olivia's class members came marching towards them; she rolled her eyes as their puerile grins spread across their faces.

"Is this your boyfriend, Alex?" they giggled, turning around at one another.

"Eurgh, what's that on your face?"

the one girl snorted, bringing attention to Jake. Immediately he covered his face with his long hair and looked down at the floor; Olivia felt outraged and seethed.

"Why don't you sort out your own insecurities? You all devote your time taunting and jeering to make yourselves feel better. Insulting people's appearance or intelligence won't improve your own. You should be ashamed of yourselves." Olivia snapped. She turned away from them, leaving the group to walk away in silence.

Jake raised his eyebrows, "That was incredible."

"I hate ignorance." she shook her head. "I get bullied and I've never found the courage to stand up for myself before but this has been a perfect opportunity to stand up for me as well as you and others who are different from those who consider themselves to be untouchable. I will be more assertive from now on."

"Me too." Jake smiled.

Olivia and Jake returned to the picture.

"What makes that picture so incredible is its hidden beauty and once people see that, they can appreciate it more." Olivia commented.

"I suppose you're right." Jake nodded. He turned towards Olivia and pushed back his hair, revealing his face again.

Olivia looked down at her wristwatch and saw it was almost four o'clock; she groaned and slung her bag over her shoulder,

"I have to go back now." she tiptoed to hug her friend and headed back towards the coach but just before she did, she handed Jake her hair bobble.

"Here." she said, "Don't hide your face anymore."

Amongst the group of people standing by the coach, she noticed the people from the gallery who taunted her and Jake; they shamefacedly glanced at Olivia before looking at their feet. Olivia finally felt assertive enough to walk with her head high for once.

A sea of heads eventually filled the coach; Olivia saw her empty seat at the back and halted.

"I will start being more assertive." she thought. She spotted the spare seat positioned to the left of her and slid onto it.

"Hi, I'm Olivia." she introduced herself to the girl sitting beside her; Olivia's heart raced yet she remained bold.

"I know." the girl replied. Olivia was taken aback. However a smile appeared as she added, "I'm Selene, pleased to meet you."

FIVE MAGIC WEEKS OF
SUMMER

Training for their circus act in the first

week of summer, a magician produced

a rabbit out of a hat,

"That wasn't what I expected!" she

laughed out loud, "Would you imagine

that?"

One by one the performers joined,

putting their tricks to the test,

"These weeks will be so exciting; we

will be our best!"

The following week another member

joined the magnificent, magical crew,

Letting out a smile, taming a crocodile,

she said "How do you do?"

A lion roared, which silenced them all,

and there stood the giant brute;

Then a mouse scuttled in, wearing a

huge grin, but the creature was

incredibly mute.

One member went missing in the third

week of summer; the lion was licking

her paws,

"I've had my lunch!" she laughed

behind the cage bars, showing her

shiny claws.

The jugglers ran, along with the tallest

man, and they all sounded the alarm,

"Don't worry" the mouse said,

"Hurray!" they applauded, feeling
rewarded, showing an enormous smile.
The three magicians fought off the
bullies with words so valiant without
rage,
"Let's put on a show!" said the one
hero, and so the three performed on
stage.

DECEPTIVE MIRROR

As I look in the mirror there's a large,
unsightly image staring back at me.
Nauseous and disgusted, I wonder how
I've gotten into this circumstance;
Only my careless doings have created
my new form along with these voices
in my head.
Reminding and hissing at me, eating
into my mind until I've convinced
myself I'm fat.
Eventually I eschewed my food; I
can't bear to put that poison to my lips.

X is what I mark on my diary, another day achieved; I will get rid of this weight.

I will be thinner. I will be beautiful. However looking at the grotesque reflection and pulling angrily at the skin on my body, I find both impossible.

And then I tell my six stone self to do it all again tomorrow, for I am monstrous, overweight and deceived.

NON

"Non-Epileptic Attack Disorder, Mrs
Jones." the doctor said,
"Non?" Mrs Jones replied, her face
glowing red,
"That word is an insult!" she started
with rage,
"Let me explain!" he said, hoping
she'd seize this rampage,
"Non-Epileptic Attack Disorder is a
seizure which doesn't attack the
brain."
She turned and asked, "So why doesn't

it have its own name?"

The lady looked at the doctor in her

green dress and pink lipstick,

And sighed, "Non makes the condition

sound extremely pessimistic."

Before the doctor could speak the lady

spoke on,

Shook her head and folded her arms

and didn't stop until she'd won.

"Not only is it comparing it to a

condition that it is not,

Its name sounds so unappealing, unlike

the other lot;

You don't get Non-colds if you have

the flu, or Non-sprains if you've

broken bones."

The doctor nodded and replied,

"You're right Mrs Jones!"

"Non means not, which implies it's
unreal,

And if you had this disorder, how
would you feel?

To say it's NOT something, rather than
it is,

And being asked questions by doctors
like some sort of quiz!"

The man in the coat uncrossed his
arms and sat upright,

And realised Mrs Jones' speech was in
fact right!

"Mrs Jones, I understand, it is truly
absurd,

This word is a trouble-maker, a truly
horrible word!

The condition's separate from epilepsy
so why is it in the name?
Even though they look alike, both
disabilities aren't the same!"
The doctor shook her hand, "I hope
you didn't take offense!"
"Well!" replied the lady, "The word is
simply NON-sense."

IGNORANT PEOPLE

There are so many people who don't
understand,
Who stare and watch without lending a
hand,
That would rather buy designer jeans
than donate a token,
To charities and events that go
unspoken,
For disabilities, whether visible or
unnoticed,
Or various mental health disorders;
neither should be dismissed,

Ignorant people think they are the
hierarchy, the noble holding their
crown,
The art of deception from the foolish;
ironic how every joke comes from a
clown,
Ignorance is for the ignorant,
uneducated and impolite;
More compassionate people will mean
less ignorance in sight.

❖

THE ELEVENTH OF OCTOBER

❖

Twelve degrees, blurred trees,

A couple's disagreement; a bus goes

by.

Stop at a red light, autumn muggy

daylight

Another ambulance with a siren rushes

by.

An old memory, reaching the

cemetery,

Three school children walking by.

Concerned dad, the radio stations not

too bad,

This road is bare; no one's walking by.

Almost home, I can't wait to be alone,

A family of three finally walk on by.

Finally here, wiping away a tear,

I think of the appointment with the

doctor, that promising guy.

HOPE, FAITH AND JOY

Three women lived in a small humble town. They each had optimistic outlooks on life which made their friendship extra special; Hope was a dreamer, who liked to wish positive things, whereas Faith was a firm believer who'd trust her instincts, and Joy was a peaceful, innocuous lady who enjoyed keeping everyone happy. However, one Tuesday afternoon Hope went missing.

"Where's Hope?" Joy asked Faith

as she approached her on her lawn. She paused for a moment before replying.

"I don't know. In fact I haven't seen her all morning!" they both looked at one another and headed towards Hope's cottage.

"Hello?" Joy shouted. They knocked on her door, waiting for their friend to appear, yet nothing happened; Faith peeked through the netted curtains only to see Hope's ginger cat curled up at the back of the chair.

"Hope?" Faith called through the letterbox; they became more worried as nobody came and so the two stood in complete silence.

"Something is wrong and we need to investigate."

Faith paced up and down as she pondered "I've got it! She usually takes a walk in the forest on Tuesday mornings to pick apples for her pies!"

"Let's go to the forest then." Joy suggested. As they trod over twisted roots and walked in amongst the wild flowers, they began to search for their friend, hoping to find her picking apples. They soon stopped as they stood before a thousand trees.

"What do we do now?" Joy sighed, gazing at the plethora of trees. "She could be anywhere!" It was as though they'd given up on their search for

Hope before it had already begun.

"Well, I'll go this way" Faith sighed pointing down the hill that slowly turned to darkness, "And you shall look that way."

Joy looked towards the friendlier route full of birds that delicately twittered and rays of sunlight that formed a well-lit path.

As they separated, Joy gradually felt more scared and lonely; the beautiful path transformed into a place that was dismal and wretched. She glanced over her shoulder warily as the birds squawked heavily and frantically flapped their wings; Joy was perplexed at how different everything appeared;

the further from Faith she got, the more miserable the place seemed.

"I don't like this." she muttered to herself, folding her arms tightly. Joy looked back and saw she was totally lost; the trees had swallowed up her existence, leaving her disorientated.

Faith walked down the hill, entering into the pit of darkness; her strong posture retreated into a hunched position as she began to feel more vulnerable.

"Hope!" her voice pierced through the silence; wishing they hadn't have parted ways, she continued to tread through crunchy leaves and the thick mud. Suddenly she found herself in complete darkness. She looked around and noticed there weren't any more trees; only extensive land and dead plants.

A heavy layer of darkness obscured her vision making her struggle to see in front. Faith unexpectedly tripped over a jagged rock, leaving her to fall further down the hill.

"Help!" she gasped, grazing her knees and arm; as she started to weep she heard a faint muffle and her ears perked. She slowly stood up and stepped forward, following the noise, wary yet intrigued.

"Hope?" Faith looked stunned. She halted and saw a woman's silhouette sitting on the ground.

"Faith!" she sighed with relief and ran towards her. "How did you know I was here?"

"I had an inkling." she shrugged. "We have to find Joy. She's looking for you too!" as they staggered up the hill the darkness eventually seized.

Throughout their mission they noticed their moods deteriorating, making them feel disheartened and empty, in Joy's absence. Faith's makeup began to leak as tears formed down her face whilst Hope moped alongside her. Although their moods were sullied, they remained ambitious about their own optimistic outlooks;

even more so as they stayed together.

"She has to be over there. I just know it!" Faith pointed; Hope agreed as they wandered into the specific region. Soon enough they heard a faint cry and they were certain it was their friend.

"Joy!" Hope and Faith exclaimed. Joy spun around and saw the two ladies sprinting towards her.

"I thought you'd never find me!" She squealed with happiness. "I almost gave up!" she saw how upset Hope and Faith were and wrapper her arms around them.

"We were so miserable without you, Joy!" Faith announced finally showing a smile, "But we didn't give up. We knew you would be here; I had a hunch."

"I wasn't terribly sad. I began to get frightened and thought you wouldn't find me out here in the woods!" Joy responded. As they looked around them, the forest had transformed into the peaceful environment they once knew full of apple trees and pretty violets that dotted about the grass.

"Let's head home." Hope saw the pathway through the surrounding trees and lead the way until they eventually reached their homes; Hope courteously asked her friends inside and they spent the evening telling tales about the incident, laughing and joking as they knew they were fortunate to escape danger.

The women's strong relationship enabled them to strengthen their emotions and sensibility and they came to the conclusion that without Joy, Hope or Faith their wellbeing would fall apart.

They laughed at their realisation and agreed never to go wandering off alone.

"Oh no!" Hope shrieked. "My apples! They must have fallen as I got lost." She shrugged her shoulders, "I'll just have to get some more tomorrow."

"Ahem!" Joy looked at Hope, reminding her of their promise.

"I mean we shall get some more tomorrow!"

THE PARCEL DELIVERY MAN

❖

"Have a nice day." he smiled, handing over a small parcel; I closed the door and watched the parcel delivery man walk down the street, swinging his keys to and fro in his hand.

His smile wasn't held long enough; his insincerity made me feel as though I had said something offensive.

He stood too close to the door invading my proximity whilst clenching his fists, blaming the cold weather, yet I knew he wanted to hit me.

He commented about the breakable item as he handed over the box. The word 'breakable' was printed out in red ink. Mocking and undermining me as he paraphrased such blatancy.

He withheld my address information as I signed for the parcel; he will return unexpectedly and harm me in unthinkable ways and deface my car as he scratches the key down its side.

Persuaded that he has returned to his station to conspire, I resume to my bedroom and look at my bed, knowing tonight's going to be forever sleepless thanks to paranoia.

THE MISSING PIECE

"Who's he?" the girl pointed to the man in the gold frame. Douglas turned round and smiled,

"My Granddad, Ted." the boy hoisted himself up from the chair and went to fetch the photograph that stood proudly on the shelf next to the porcelain ornaments; he studied it for a second before handing it over to his friend who was intrigued to find out more.

"He has a lovely smile." she

immediately noticed at how pleasant and jovial he appeared. "How old is he?"

"He was eighty-nine there." he nodded before returning the photo to the shelf. Silence erupted before another question about his granddad came from his friend,

"How old is he now?" she wondered, raising her eyebrows; she thought his incredible age with his youthful appearance seemed somewhat paradoxical.

The boy slowly sat in his original position and hesitated.

"He passed away last March." he crumbled into a forlorn state as he reflected, "He had dementia." his brief eye contact with his friend allowed her to see how painful the final memories were for him and so she deferred from the topic.

"Where was that photo taken anyway?" she glanced back at the tall man holding a cocktail glass under a parasol.

"Spain" a smile started to crack and slightly show, "he would go there quite a lot."

As this encouraged a light-hearted conversation, she continued asking more, "What was he like?"

Immediately his eyes glinted and he sat up straight, smiling as he spoke about the happier memories of his granddad.

"He was really independent and wouldn't let you do anything for him; he was always on the go as well" as he stared into thin air it was as though he was reinventing the memories and watching them play before his eyes like an old video with a projector. "He always kept himself fit and healthy, I suppose that was because he was in the army, but he would always go to the shops and fetch a newspaper and do exercises – even at the age of ninety!"

His friend gasped, looking amazed, "That is amazing!" she pleaded to know more about Ted; she found his stories fascinating and so she sat comfortably in her chair and waited for another story to conjure up.

"He was a practical joker too- he had a great sense of humour and I remember we went to a Christmas party and he tied his friend's shoe laces together!" he laughed and his friend showed a wide smile; his expression dropped as he remembered his condition made an appearance shortly after.

"What's wrong?" his friend asked placing her head in her hand; he turned towards her and pouted lowering his tone.

"It was a few days after that we

noticed he started acting a little different...not like him" she tilted her head to the side, predicting the light-hearted story to plummet into an unhappy one.

"How?"

"Well he stopped eating; skipping meals and so he lost loads of weight."

The cheery man was a healthy size but Douglas pictured a frailer man that sat before him on his regular visits.

"Deliberately?" his friend quizzed; her eyes grew wide with concern.

"Sometimes we had to force him to have food because he didn't want to eat and he had to. Then he just started forgetting to." he said bluntly, "Some days he would tell us that he had eaten but I could guess that it was probably untrue. I would find food in the bin that hadn't been touched." unsure whether he would continue, his friend gazed at him, contemplating changing the subject.

However, he pulled his mouth the side and continued to speak about his granddad's hardest times.

"Some days he was more himself though but that was rare; I remember he had fixations on things, which was one of the reasons why we took him to the doctors." he saw her eyebrows shift downwards with both sincerity and interest. "He accused my brother of stealing his gold watch the once; he hadn't but he was adamant that it had been taken."

"What happened at the doctors then? What did they do?" her face looked focused.

"They put him on medication called Citalopram, a well-known anti-depressant, but it helped with his Dementia too as well as his depression."

He stood up suddenly and excused himself before running out of the room; his friend placed her hands together and waited patiently for him to return, assuming Douglas had gotten too upset about it.

Moments after he re-entered holding a large red book with the pages peeping slightly out of the bottom.

"Here." he smiled, folding the leather cover back to reveal a photograph sellotaped to the page.

Douglas and his friend scrutinised each photo whilst he told a story that was significant about him; she smiled, listening to how thoughtful he was towards him.

As they flicked the pages she noticed his Granddad maintained a very stylish appearance with neatly combed hair.

"He was very handsome." she

mentioned, "He dressed very well too!"

"Yes, well, he did dress very smart but that was another thing – he stopped looking after himself a bit because of his condition." she nodded at his words,

"I suppose that's understandable though; he may have gotten annoyed at his condition. Was he aware that his memory was getting worse?"

"He was at first; he knew something wasn't right but he refused to admit to it. Then it got to the stage where he'd become confused with faces and names and he was unaware of his behaviour. It's a neurodegenerative disease so it doesn't ever get better." he paused before adding, "I remember he'd look at me sometimes; he was very unsure to whom I was and sometimes he'd call my dad Peter, which was my Granddad's brother's name."

They turned another page to reveal a sepia coloured picture with his wife, who was wearing a skirt that reached the knee with an elegant blouse with flowers; they both looked in their thirties and as pleasant as each other.

"That's my nan, Sarah. She was lovely." her shoulder length curly hair framed her face perfectly; the couple complemented each other and they happily stood in front of a black nineteen-forty's Ford. "That car was my granddad's prize possession; he'd drive it everywhere but he stopped when he reached his late sixties."

"Was that due to his illness?" Douglas' friend asked.

"Oh no, he was just a very cautious and responsible person in that respect; he thought his driving wasn't so brilliant anymore and was becoming a danger to others on the road and so he stopped driving. He was also very careful as he would always worry about drinks spilling or vases breaking and so he'd just make sure they were neatly secured in places where they couldn't be."

One of the most significant traits Douglas' granddad started to display during the eighteen months of his condition was his carelessness; he would become more accepting to people's help, whereas before he'd wait patiently on them, instead he'd sometimes make situations more cumbersome.

As pages turned, Douglas halted at a specific page as he had found his favourite picture.

"This was for granddad's ninetieth birthday!" the picture showed a large sum of people surrounding his Granddad each wearing birthday hats and wide smiles. "That's my mother and father, my aunties and uncles, my cousins and that's me." he pointed to each member, recapping how marvellous that day was, and then he let out a laugh.

"What's so funny?" his friend quizzed. She saw him point to a pine table that lay in front of him with a jigsaw puzzle splayed out on it.

"He lost just one piece from that puzzle and always said it would turn up, but it never did! He remembered that missing jigsaw puzzle better than he did most things!"

"Was his memory always bad?" she asked, still studying the

photograph's happy faces.

"Strangely he remembered certain things, such as his long term memory; he could tell you things from what happened years ago but his short term memory was terrible! He would forget quite a lotand it would make him so confused at times!"

They finished the book with the most recent photo of his granddad; Douglas' friend soon realised how much of an impact his condition had on himself as well as his family members and friends. His appearance, such as his hair, wasn't as neat anymore and his shirts were unkempt.

Also, his frame had changed

dramatically from rotund to slightly gaunt.

"He looks so much different!" she commented; Douglas nodded, avoiding eye contact.

"Let's have a break from this!" Douglas suddenly announced; the revisiting memories were almost too much for Douglas to continue at the present moment. "Would you like a drink?"

As they headed towards the kitchen Douglas' friend couldn't help but notice more photographs of his Granddad dotted around on shelves and walls.

"You were very fond of him,

weren't you?" she smiled; again Douglas nodded and poured some juice into a couple of glasses.

The sunny afternoon gave a soothing presence; they sat in the garden and relaxed, appreciating the warmth. As the girl looked over at Douglas, she noticed he was staring intently at the picture of his Granddad with the jigsaw puzzle that he'd taken out of the photo album.

"What's wrong?" she queried; his eyes were fixated on the tiny photograph and after a moment of silence he let out a hearty laugh.

"Do you see this?" he pointed to the picture. She tilted her head with confusion,

"Yes. You have already shown me."

"Look behind him!" he grinned; as she scrutinised the picture, something became more apparent; it was the missing piece to the jigsaw! "It's wedged at the back of the box!"

They both laughed for a minute before his friend turned towards him,

"Where is he?" looking at the surroundings with the pine coffee table and lilac walls.

"He's at his residential home in this photo. I used to visit him every day after school. It was depressing going there but my granddad needed support;

even though I felt he wasn't so much like my granddad anymore." he paused and looked back at his friend, who looked as though she was thinking.

"Let's go back and see if it's still there!" she spoke in an excited manner, "There's no guarantee it will still be there but it's worth a try!"

The friends immediately slipped their shoes and coats on and started their journey; it had been a while since Douglas had visited yet he remembered it all so well.

As they reached the residential home, Douglas' friend stopped and looked up at the white building.

"It's beautiful!" the neatly cut

garden lay around the side with a plethora of benches for the residents to sit and enjoy the water features or birds flittering about and a stony path that lead all the way to the entrance.

"Hi I'm Douglas Wiltshore" he introduced himself to the receptionist who he saw almost every day, "I was Theodore Wiltshore's grandson."

The woman's eyebrows rose and she released a pleasant smile, "I remember Teddy!" she replied, "He was lovely bloke. What can I do for you?" she sat there with her biro in her hand and waited for his preposterous reply.

"I was wondering whether we

could visit his room." the lady pouted and shook her head.

"I'm ever so sorry but someone else lives there now!" Douglas looked at the floor anticipating that response.

"Come on." his friend smiled, "At least we tried." as she turned round she noticed something glint; a small blue plastic object that perfectly matched the jigsaw piece in the photo. She nudged Douglas and pointed towards the object on the shelf with stacks of books tightly packed.

"That's it!" he looked in disbelief. As they walked over, the object became more apparent and it was the exact piece his granddad was missing.

"*How can this be?*" Douglas thought. Both of them were amazed; it was as though fate had awarded them the opportunity to find the piece.

Douglas picked up the tiny object and clasped it in his hand; his friend and the receptionist turned to him, marvelling at how delighted he was.

"Excuse me, does this mean anything to you?" he questioned, adamant that the piece was a victim of the lost and found; the receptionist laughed.

"That must have fallen out of the book!" the slender lady pointed to the book behind the item, which gained their attention. They slid the hardback out from the others and saw it was a personal book dedicated to a Mr. Theodore Wiltshore.

Douglas and his friend's face lit up; all of the books were personalised and devoted to a resident that once lived here. As they opened the book, their eyes grew wide as they saw an overabundance of comments from his family and friends, commenting on what a marvellous man he was.

"Look!" his friend gasped as she pointed to a particular statement; it stated:

"To a dear friend, here is the missing piece."

They both smiled and swiftly

Douglas asked the receptionist,

"May I take this piece?" he held out the object and awaited her response.

The lady looked at the boy's over-zealous expression and took a deep breath,

"As you are his grandson, I don't see why not!" she paused for a second, "Why though?"

As Douglas planted it in his pocked he announced with a wide grin,

"My granddad said it would always turn up, and here it is, so I would like to put it with the rest of the puzzle!"

The receptionist laughed, "Ted was always making that comment to us;

when we found it we decided to put it alongside the comments in his memorial book. Funny isn't it how little things get remembered like that?" Douglas nodded as they turned away, heading back home.

Later on that day they slid out the dusty jigsaw box from above the wardrobe; it was a bare room that hadn't been used in a few years.

"Let's finish this puzzle!" Douglas' friend said, fetching out the pieces. That evening the friends shared more stories about Theodore Wiltshire and once the missing piece slotted in between the picture, it was finally complete.

Douglas fetched his Polaroid camera and took a photo of the masterpiece; once the picture had developed he placed it in front of him and his friend.

"Perfect!" she stated, feeling an overwhelming sense of achievement.

"I think this completes it, don't you?" they meandered into the lounge, where they were originally seated, and opened the book up once more.

"Here you go, Granddad!" Douglas said quietly; he sellotaped the recent picture onto the last page.

"The missing piece." his friend voiced, "The most important I think."

"How so?" Douglas asked; she held

the book in both hands and gazed upon the completed album,

"That things always return to you. Old things can become new again- just like his stories!"

Douglas let out a laugh, "I suppose you're right!"

Theodore's anecdotes had put the couple into high spirits and they realised that not all memories were forgotten. In fact they could be renewed as many times as they wished.

Finally he fetched out a biro and marked the page next to the photograph whilst smiling and entitled it *The missing piece*.

BORDERLINE

On the verge, on the edge,

With my relationships I've driven a

wedge.

I don't mean to as it's not me;

It's deep within so you can't see.

It leaves me thinking and behaving as

such,

The stress, the feeling, is all too much.

Distorted and worthless is all I think,

Suicide attempts on the brink.

My body says two things: "I love you"

from the heart,

"Get away" Says the condition, which
pushes us apart.
But the key to making my head clear,
To make this illness disappear;
Is the medication; it's an effective
way,
To keep this specific lifestyle at bay;
To banish this disorder and get on with
my life
Instead of feeling angst and torment
whilst holding a knife.
My head feels clearer and I feel fine,
I'm in control of this personality
disorder they call 'Borderline'.

TWO SIDES TO THE STORY

One extreme to the other,

One phase to another,

It's something that is really absurd.

Hard to get your head around it,

Or even just a little bit,

As this condition is seen but never

heard.

For people who are clueless,

Even for people who know this,

I'll reiterate the facts so you know;

There's mania and depression,

And this is the valuable lesson:

Bipolar moods swing to and fro.

With mania, you experience euphoria,

That high feeling of superior,

Although it can spiral into something

worse.

With Depression you feel the opposite,

Feeling like you're in a bottomless pit,

That you're worthless; these symptoms

are quite diverse!

For each person this condition

modifies,

Either by longer downs or shorter

highs,

It's not always as dramatic as you

think.

Some people may have excessive

pride,

Some people think about suicide;

This mental illness pushes you to the

brink!

So when people suddenly recognise,

The condition's not such a surprise,

Everyone understands and an ear they

lend.

For this risky behaviour,

You could be their saviour,

A person that you can call a friend.

IT'S IN THE BLOOD

Jimmy: I've been reading up on Leukaemia. Did you know it's a type of cancer?

Dylan: I'm impressed! Tell me more…

Jimmy: Well, it's cancer of the blood; it affects certain blood cells but particularly the white blood cells, also known as Leukocytes, which are there to protect the body and fight off infections!

Dylan: Wow you have been reading!

Jimmy: Do you know there's more than one type of Leukaemia? They are categorised into: Chronic and Acute stages.

Dylan: What can you tell me about that?

Jimmy: In acute Leukaemia the "immature" leukocytes, which are normally found in bone marrow, accumulates; this is a problem for the tissue and organ functions in the body! Examples of Acute Leukaemia are: Acute Lymphoblastic Leukaemia and Acute Myeloid Leukaemia.

Dylan: What are they then?

Jimmy: Acute Lymphoblastic Leukaemia is when you have an overabundance of immature white leukocytes; they continuously multiply and are overproduced in the bone marrow. Acute Myeloid Leukaemia is also cancer that starts inside the soft tissue inside bones we call bone marrow. In fact, Myeloid Leukaemia is the most common types amongst adults!

Dylan: How about examples of chronic Leukaemia?

Jimmy: Well there's Chronic Lymphocytic Leukaemia and Chronic Myeloid Leukaemia; Chronic Lymphocytic Leukaemia and Chronic Myeloid Leukaemia is when the body has an abnormal increase of mature lymphocytes, which is also a type of white blood cell; unlike the acute cases where they are more aggressive and progress faster, these take longer to progress, taking symptoms longer to develop.

Dylan: I am impressed! You seem to have grasped it.

Jimmy: I think I have. I spent all last night reading about it!

Dylan: I bet you're tired!

Jimmy: Well did you know fatigue is a symptom of Leukaemia?

Dylan: I did, but would you care to tell me more about the symptoms?

Jimmy: Well if generalised weakness and fatigue wasn't enough there are lots more, such as anaemia where there's not enough healthy blood cells, making the person pale, and again, tired.

Dylan: That's awful. Anything else?

Jimmy: Oh yes! Bleeding, excessive bruising, frequent infections such as fevers, pain in the joints and bones…

Dylan: That is a lot!

Jimmy: There's more: breathlessness, headaches, weight loss, seizures, enlarged lymph nodes which are also sore to the touch and vomiting too!

Dylan: Unimaginable. What causes Leukaemia?

Jimmy: It is not known in most cases, but some factors are: being exposed to high levels of radiation, smoking, family history, age, or exposure to benzene; all of these can increase the risk of Leukaemia but the different factors depend on the type of leukaemia.

Dylan: I see.

Jimmy: It is also the twelfth most common cancer in the UK; with a forty-five per cent survival rate at least five years after diagnoses and around 4,500 deaths in the UK a year.

Dylan: That's twelve people per day!

Jimmy: I may read up on something else; I think I am getting the hang of remembering things.

Dylan: Yes I'm sure you have! Did

you remember to take the book back to the library?

Jimmy: Oops! I forgot…

About the author

Sophiedallaway.wix.com/books

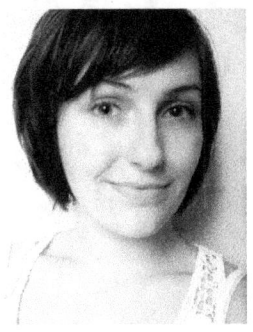

Sophie Dallaway is an English poet and author who trained as a nurse in 2009. Sophie has a passion for health care and medicine and aspires to work with patients with dementia as well as other illnesses. Hopefully this book will raise awareness of various disabilities and conditions that so many people are unaware of.

Thank you for reading Brainstorming!

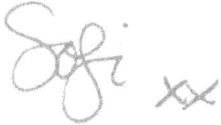

www.ingramcontent.com/pod-product-compliance
Lightning Source LLC
Chambersburg PA
CBHW071341280526
45787CB00001B/173